Gluten Free

Gluten free for beginners, and how to live the gluten free lifestyle including gluten free diet, paleo, gluten free benefits, and more!

Table Of Contents

Introduction

I want to thank you and congratulate you for downloading the book, "Gluten Free".

This book contains helpful information about the Gluten free lifestyle, and the benefits of living Gluten free.

A Gluten free diet is great for your health. It can help you lose weight, and also naturally increase your energy levels.

A Gluten free, or Paleo style diet is what our bodies are naturally suited to, thanks to human evolution over the last several million years. As a result, many people experience health complications and feel lethargic thanks to Gluten in their diet.

You will soon learn exactly what the Gluten free diet is, how you can begin adopting this diet, and the great range of benefits it can provide.

This book will explain to you tips and techniques that will allow you to begin successfully improving your health with a gluten free diet today! For your ease of application, this book also includes several delicious Gluten free recipes that will help to get you started!

So read on, and begin implementing the Gluten free diet and lifestyle today!

Thanks again for downloading this book. I hope you enjoy it!

Chapter 1:
Benefits of Gluten Free Diet

The gluten free diet has become very popular because of its numerous benefits, especially for those with certain health conditions. Gluten is a protein that is normally found in wheat and barley. People who have Celiac disease or those who suffer from gluten sensitivity need to follow the gluten free diet to avoid serious health complications.

Going Gluten Free and The Paleo Diet

Gluten free diet and Paleo diet share some similarities. The main reason that most people switch to gluten free diet is their food intolerances. The Paleo diet carries many health benefits including a reduction in the risk of heart disease, cancer and diabetes. Paleo diet is also often paired with several workout regimens and is used in weight loss programs.

The Gluten free and Paleo diet emphasizes on the consumption of whole foods. Paleo diet in particular forbids the consumption of any food that was not consumed during the Paleolithic age, which includes sugar, wheat and artificial additives. Eliminating processed foods from your diet will drastically increase your energy levels and improve your physical and mental health.

The main benefit derived from Gluten free and Paleo diets largely depends on your motivation for making the diet switch. If you choose to live a gluten free lifestyle because of food intolerance and Celiac disease, the main benefit that you will experience is relief from the symptoms. However, there are also people who choose to follow a gluten free lifestyle for non-medical reasons.

Benefits of Gluten Free & Paleo Diet

Better Digestion

People who suffer from digestive problems can greatly benefit from a gluten free diet. Gluten can cause inflammation in the intestines for people with Celiac disease. Gluten can also reduce the amount of nutrients absorbed in the body which can lead to lack of energy and malnutrition. People who switch to a gluten free diet can reduce the risk of bloating, gas, constipation and stomach cramps.

Inflammation

People who suffer from gluten intolerance can also suffer from joint pain and numb legs. A gluten free or Paleo diet can reduce skin and muscle inflammation. Studies also show that eliminating gluten can also improve skin conditions like eczema and acne.

Improved Energy Levels

Removing processed foods that are rich in empty calories can drastically increase your energy levels. People who are sensitive to gluten are most likely unable to absorb enough vitamins and minerals which can lead to fatigue. Eating a variety or vegetables, fruits and organic meat can provide you with the energy that you will need.

Provides Detox effects

You are reducing the toxin buildup in your body by eliminating processed foods. You will also get a lot of antioxidants from vegetables and fruits which can stimulate a detoxification process in the body.

Balances blood glucose levels

A Gluten free diet can help you maintain a regular blood glucose level. It can also help you avoid fatigue and mood swings caused by blood sugar spikes. Following the gluten free diet is a better choice than the standard diet when it comes to preventing diabetes.

Non-Medical Benefits of Gluten Free Diet

Gives you a sense of accomplishment

Make a list of what you need to do in order to become healthier. This includes shopping for whole foods, preparing healthy meals and scheduling regular workouts. Making a list and ensuring that you follow it can produce a sense of fulfillment. This can make you feel good and improve your self-esteem.

Reduces health care cost

Maintaining a healthy diet is one of the best things that you can do to ensure that you live a long and fruitful life. A healthy and clean diet is like an investment in the long run. An overall healthy lifestyle can help you avoid expensive medical treatments in the future.

Makes you look younger

Living a healthy lifestyle can make you look younger. Vegetables and fruits are rich in antioxidants that can help reduce oxidative stress in the body. It also protects the cells from free radicals and can result in fresh and glowing skin. Whole foods also promote cell regeneration which can make your skin look smooth and supple.

Live a long and fulfilled life

One of the advantages of switching to a healthy diet is that you are able to enjoy different activities more often. You can become more productive during the day and it can also help you become more positive. Supplementing your diet with regular exercise and stress reduction can enable you to live your life to the fullest.

Chapter 2:
Gluten Free Diet Basics

The concept of the Gluten free diet has been introduced during the past few years. Below are the basics of the Gluten Free and Paleo diet.

Gluten Free Diet Basics:

Use whole foods

Some people may not want to shift to a gluten free diet because they think that it is too restrictive. Contrary to popular belief, there are a lot of foods that you can consume while on a gluten free diet. Focus on whole foods like fruits, vegetables and meat.

The Paleo diet in particular encourages the consumption of beef, lamb, organ meat and seafood. Meat is a rich source of protein and healthy fats. Eating enough protein can also help you lose weight and build lean muscle. You should also consume different colored vegetables.

Use a flour substitute

You do not have to avoid baked goods entirely. You can use healthier flour substitutes like coconut flour, almond flour and tapioca flour. These flour substitutes are made with complex carbohydrates that are rich in nutrients. They can also add texture and unique flavor to your food. Try experimenting with healthy fillings like fruits, herbs and spices instead of sugar.

Focus on nutrients, not just calories

Do not get too caught up in the number of calories that you are consuming. Most people are too focused on the calorie-in and calorie-out approach in order to lose weight. However, counting calories isn't exactly healthy. 200 calories of green smoothie is still a better choice than a zero calorie soda. Remember that getting enough of the right nutrients is better than counting calories.

Control your sugar consumption

People are usually unaware of their total sugar consumption. Sugar is added to processed foods and most restaurants serve meals that are full of added sugar. The recommended sugar consumption for women is only 6 teaspoons while men should only have 9 teaspoons of sugar per day. Opt for natural sweeteners like honey or maple syrup instead. You can drastically reduce your sugar consumption by eliminating soda, candy and processed breads. Also, some healthy foods like flavored yogurt have added sugar so opt for the plain variety instead.

Totally giving up sweet treats may seem impossible for some people who have a particular affinity to sweet foods. Fruits are great alternative to candy bars. Their natural sweetness can curb your cravings, and they can also provide you with fiber and nutrients. You can also make your own desserts and treats using whole ingredients.

Use healthy fats

Vegetable oil does not actually come from vegetables. It contains large amounts of Omega 6 fatty acid that can be harmful for your health in large doses. Fortunately, there are a lot of healthy fats to choose from when it comes to a Gluten free diet. You can use animal fat like lard, bacon fat and tallow. Coconut oil and olive oil are also popular alternatives.

Follow the 80/20 rule

While some people may opt for the 'all of nothing' approach, it is actually unrealistic to follow. Following the 80/20 rule means that you consume an 80% gluten free diet while giving yourself enough space to indulge in occasional treats. Switching to a completely different diet can take some time. Make sure that you make room for adjustments so that you will not be depressed when you experience a setback. However, this rule is only applicable for people who are switching to gluten free diet for non-medical purposes. People who suffer from Celiac and food intolerance must absolutely avoid gluten at all cost or they may experience dangerous consequences.

Read the label

Gluten, wheat and sugar are usually added in most processed foods. Make sure that you always read the label of the food item that you are buying. Fortunately, there are a lot of organic, natural and gluten free stores and companies that sell healthier alternatives to commercial products.

Remember that there may be companies that label their food as 'gluten-free' or 'wheat-free'. The food and drug administration requires all products that are labeled as 'gluten-free' to contain less than 20 parts of gluten. Products that are labeled as 'wheat-free' can still contain gluten. As a general rule, if you are not sure if the product contains gluten, don't buy it or check with the manufacturer first.

Watch out for cross contamination

Cross contamination is common when you live in a household where not everyone follows the diet. Cross contamination can happen when you use the same kitchen and food utensils for both gluten and gluten-free food. For example, you use the same knife to spread butter into your bread then use the same knife to cut your vegetables. To avoid this, make sure that you clean utensils after each use. You can also label ingredients to avoid confusion.

Other Lifestyle Tips to Complement a Gluten Free Diet:

Don't forget to move

One disadvantage of having a modern lifestyle is that people don't get enough exercise. Being sedentary can be easy with the convenience of technology. Aside from a healthy diet, you also need to make sure that you are getting enough exercise. There are many forms of exercise to choose from so it will be easy to find something that can suit your preference.

Improve your sleep

Sleep is a human necessity and not a luxury. You will also be more productive after a good night sleep. Settle down and do relaxing activities in the evening so that you can sleep better at night.

Get outdoors

Your workplace or home may be more comfortable than the hills and mountains, but it is also important to get some fresh air and see the beautiful sights that Mother Nature has to offer. There are many studies that show the positive results of getting in touch with nature and spending time outdoors. It can help you relax and unwind as well as improve your mood.

Chapter 3:
Make Maintaining the Gluten Free Diet Easy

Clean eating can be convenient if you know how to plan your meals. Here are some tips on how you can make meal preparation much easier:

Set time to make your own packed foods

Chopping and washing vegetables can take some time especially if you do it on a daily basis. Set a few hours during the weekend to prepare most of your foods for the following week. If you don't like to spend a long time cooking your breakfast in the morning, then you can create your own granola mixture and store it in the refrigerator. You can also cook foods and place them in individual serving containers and store them in the refrigerator.

Invest in Mason jars

Mason jars are very versatile. You can use these jars to store spices, condiments and small fruits. You can also layer your salad in the jar and keep it in the refrigerator. Take it to work with you and dump the contents in a bowl or eat straight from the jar. The glass jar keeps your lettuce crisp and fresh even after a week. The trick is to pour the dressing at the bottom of the jar and layer in juicy fruits and vegetables like tomatoes and cucumber before you top them with lettuce leaves. The tomatoes and cucumber act as a barrier so that the lettuce remains dry. Mason jars can withstand high temperatures so you can bake pancakes and treats in your jar. Storing your meals in mason jars also helps you control your serving size and prevents you from overeating.

Opt for a shake

Most people find it difficult to consume five servings of fruits and vegetables per day. Blending your fruits and vegetables is a convenient way to complete your daily requirement of fresh produce.

The main difference between a juice and a smoothie is that the nutrients and fiber are retained in the smoothie because the skin of the fruit and vegetable is included in the drink. You can also make green smoothies as your pre or post workout drink.

Make your own snacks

You can bake cookies using alternative flours and serve them as snacks or desserts during the entire week. Making your own snacks is more budget-friendly and convenient because it prevents you from eating junk food. You can also store ready-to-eat snacks like fruits and nuts.

Buy cheap cuts of meat and cook them in a slow cooker

Quality organic meat is the most nutritious meat in the market, but it is also possibly the most expensive meat. Learn to adjust and purchase cheap cuts of meat and cook them in a slow cooker. Cooking it for a long time tenderizes the meat and brings out its flavor. The nutrients are also preserved in the soup or casserole.

Using a slow cooker also saves you a lot of time since you only need to chop your ingredients and dump them all in the cooker. You can leave it cooking while you go to work and return to a delicious and well-cooked meal at the end of the day.

Use a food processor

How you cut your produce is important when making convenient and healthy dishes. Vegetables lose their nutrients rapidly as soon as they are cut. You can quickly chop vegetables and other produce using a food processor. It reduces the preparation time drastically. A food processor is also great to use to make meatballs, salads and sauces.

Plan in advance

Planning your weekly meals is essential to reduce the amount of food waste and to prevent last minute grocery shopping. It is a good idea to plan out your menu at least 5-7 days ahead. You can even write it down and stick it on your refrigerator to serve as a reminder. Planning your meals also helps you balance the whole foods that you are consuming. This allows you to see if you are consuming more of one produce. Planning your meals for an entire week may take some time during the week end but it will save you time during the weekdays when you are at your busiest.

Cook in huge batches

The main idea is to prepare a large batch of food that can last for a few days so that you do not have to bother cooking multiple times a day. You can freeze soups, dishes and even snacks and reheat them when you are ready to serve. This can help you save a lot of time and will help you avoid bingeing on unhealthy foods when you come home hungry and there is no healthy food available.

Chapter 4:
Going Gluten-free on a Budget

One of the misconceptions about the Gluten free diet is that you need to spend a lot of money on it. Some whole foods can be more expensive than their processed counterparts. However, you can still eat healthy and whole foods without compromising your budget. Here are some strategies for clean eating while sticking to a budget:

Set a budget and meal plan

You should set a comfortable and realistic budget. Plan your meals for a week. This provides you with a wider perspective on how you can allocate your budget. Planning your meals weekly helps you balance your diet and ensure that you are getting enough carbohydrates, protein and fat. Next, take an inventory of the ingredients in your pantry and refrigerator. List the things that you need to buy and list alternative ingredients so that you will have more options when choosing your ingredients.

Avoid packaged and pre-packed food

Convenience comes at a cost. Chopped and packed vegetables tend to cost more than the whole vegetable itself. You can buy the vegetables in bulk and chop them yourself then pack them into containers.

Shop at a local farmers market

Farmers markets usually sell organic foods cheap. You can also buy in bulk so that you don't have to shop often. You can freeze your excess food, and defrost it as you need.

Buy foods that are in season

Fruits and vegetables tend to be cheaper and are more delicious when they are in season. Learn to be flexible and incorporate them in your dishes. Fruits are great to add in pastry goods and smoothies. You can also blend green vegetables and turn them into a delicious shake.

Stock up during sales

Take advantage of sales and stock up on whole and healthy foods. You may have not included them in your weekly meal plan, but you can always freeze them or store them for later use. Dry products like grains and beans can also be safely stored in your pantry.

Limit eating out

Restaurant bills can pile up. Even regular visits to an organic or healthy restaurant can become expensive in the long run. Use your budget as a challenge and learn how to cook delicious and healthy foods. You can also invest in cookbooks and some kitchen equipment to help you get comfortable with Gluten free cooking.

Grow your greens

It can be more economical to grow your own food. You can try planting your own food if you have enough space in your backyard. Lettuce seeds can cost just $2 and you can harvest enough produce from that to last for a month. If you live in an apartment, then you can also try planting in pots. You can try planting herbs, spices and vegetables like tomatoes.

Get creative in reusing your leftovers

Do not throw leftovers out immediately. Use your creativity and incorporate them into other dishes. Meat can be sliced into strips and can be mixed with sauce to make a delicious sandwich filling. You can preserve fruits and vegetables through the canning method. You can also add vegetables to stews. You can cook foods in a large batch and freeze the extra portions.

Make your own dressing and sauces

A bottle of dressing can cost $3 and it is full of chemicals, preservatives and added sugar. An organic and natural dressing can cost twice as much. Make your own dressing using whole products and it will only cost you pennies to a dollar. This also allows you to control the ingredients.

Explore shops

Most people waste so much time wandering around in the supermarket and end up buying more than what they intend to get. Make sure that you know all food markets in your area and pay attention to markets that sell fresh and organic produce. Some stores can price their whole produce cheaper than other stores. You might also be surprised at the products offered in a small whole food market.

Transitioning to a healthy lifestyle can take some patience and sacrifice. Over time, you will learn to adjust your budget to suit your healthy lifestyle.

Chapter 5:
Sample Recipes

It's fun to experiment with different nutritious ingredients to prepare gluten free meals. Here are some sample recipes that you can try:

Butterflied Turkey with Apple Cranberry Glaze

Turkey with apple cranberry glaze is perfect to serve during special occasions. The sweet and savory glaze adds wonderful flavor to the turkey.

Ingredients:

- 1 tbsp salt

- ¼ cup coriander seeds, crushed

- 1 tsp white peppercorns

- 3 garlic cloves, smashed

- 2 tsp ground coriander

- ¾ cup honey

- 3 star anise pods

- 2 inch ginger, thinly sliced

- 12 lb turkey

For the glaze:

- 2 inch ginger, sliced

- 3 dried chili peppers

- ½ cup apple cider vinegar

- 4 tbsp cold unsalted butter, diced

- 3 cups apple cider vinegar

- 1 cup frozen cranberries

- ½ cup molasses

- Salt to taste

Makes 6-8 servings

Instructions:

1. Prepare the turkey ahead of time. Combine the honey, salt, water, star anise, peppercorns, garlic, ginger and coriander seeds in a saucepan. Let it boil over medium heat. Stir to combine the ingredients. Remove from the heat then add 4 cups of cold water.

2. Place the turkey in a container and pour the liquid over it. Refrigerate for at least 6 hours. Remove the turkey and season it with excess coriander seeds. Place in the refrigerator for 4 hours.

3. Prepare the glaze. Combine the molasses, vinegar, cranberries, ginger, chili and apple cider in a pot. Boil it over medium heat. Simmer until the liquid is thick. Whisk the mixture then strain. Season it with the salt.

4. Set the oven 375 degrees. Place the turkey on the roasting pan. Cook it for 1- 1 ½ hours. Brush the glaze on top of the turkey every 10 minutes and cook until it is brown and crispy. Remove from the heat and let it cool for 15 minutes. Grill the turkey and cook for 1 hour and 20 minutes. Brush the turkey with the glaze then serve.

Beef and Bok Choy Stir Fry

Bok choy is a common vegetable added in stir fry dishes. It has a mild flavor but is rich in nutrients. This dish is a great way to consume vegetables without knowing it.

Ingredients:

- 1 ½ lb top sirloin, thinly slices into strips

- 3 cups mushrooms, quartered

- 1 tbsp minced garlic

- Half head bok choy

- Coconut oil

For the beef marinade:

- 1 1.2 tsp arrowroot powder

- 1 tbsp tamari sauce, gluten free

- Pinch of fresh black pepper

For the sauce:

- 2 tbsp honey

- 2 tbsp arrowroot powder

- ½ cup gluten free soy sauce

- 1 tsp ground ginger

Makes 4 servings

Instructions:

1. Wash the beef and cut it into pieces. Combine the marinade ingredients in a bowl and stir. Pour it over the beef and set aside for 10 minutes.

2. Slice the bok choy and chop off the white stem. Mix the sauce ingredients in a separate bowl and set aside.

3. Place the pan over medium heat. Spread the coconut oil until melted. Once the oil is sizzling, add the beef and cook on both sides for 2-3 minutes. Make sure that you do not overcook the beef. Transfer to plate then set aside.

4. Add the mushrooms, garlic and bok choy to the pan. Stir and sauté until the bok choy is tender.

5. Add back the meat. Stir to combine. Pour the sauce over the meat. Continue to cook for 2 minutes until the sauce is thick.

Peri Peri Chicken Kebabs

Peri Peri is a Portugal dish that has the right amount of spiciness. The dish is flavored by natural spices.

Ingredients:

- 2 lb free-range organic chicken breast, cut into chunks

- Juice of 2 lemons

- 2 garlic cloves, crushed

- ½ tsp cayenne pepper

- 1 tsp oregano

- ½ tsp fine grain salt

- ½ cup white vinegar

- ¼ cup olive oil

- 1 shallot, thinly slices

- 2 tsp paprika

- 2 tsp chili powder

- Ground black pepper to taste

- Cooking spray

Makes 6 servings

Instructions:

1. Mix the lemon juice, cayenne pepper, garlic, paprika, chili powder, black pepper, oregano, salt, olive oil, shallot and white vinegar.

2. Cut the chicken into chunks then place it in a sealable bag. Pour the marinade inside. Seal and marinate for 30 minute to overnight to achieve full flavor.

3. Soak the skewer in water for 5 minutes. Remove the chicken from the bag and thread into the skewer.

4. Preheat the grill or pan. Coat the grill with cooking spray. Grill the chicken until it is cooked through and the sides are golden brown. This should take about 10 minutes.

5. Transfer to plate and serve with parsley.

Paleo Meatball Soup

This is a quick and easy soup recipe that is perfect to store in the freezer. It contains lot of vegetables and spices that provide a lot of health benefits.

Ingredients:

- 3 tbsp olive oil

- 3 celery stalks, thinly sliced

- 15 oz tomatoes, crushed

- 2 tsp oregano

- 1 tsp pepper

- 1 lb ground beef

- ¼ cup almond meal

- 1 cup broccoli

- 1 cup cauliflower

- 1 parsnip, sliced

- 1 medium onion, minced

- 2 garlic cloves, chopped

- 2 cups beef broth

- 3 tbsp fresh basil

- 1 egg

- 1 tsp garlic powder

- 3 cups baby spinach

- 1 zucchini, chopped

Makes 6 servings

Instructions:

1. Heat 3 tablespoons of oil in a pot. Add the celery and onions. Stir until it is soft and fragrant.

2. Add the garlic and cook for another minute. Add the tomatoes, broth and other vegetables except spinach. Season the dish with ½ tsp salt, 1 tsp oregano and 2 tsp basil. Simmer the mixture.

3. Make the meatballs. Combine the ground beef, 1 tsp oregano, 1 tsp pepper, almond meal, egg and 1 tbsp garlic powder in a large mixing bowl.

4. Stir the mixture using your hands. Scoop one tablespoon of the mixture and shape it into meatballs. Add the meatballs to the soup.

5. Add the spinach and remaining basil. Cook the mixture for another 20 minutes until it is cooked through.

Kelp Noodle Soup

Kelp noodles are a great substitute for wheat noodles. It is usually available in most health food stores. This noodle soup recipe is very versatile and can be prepared in a short amount of time.

Ingredients:

- 6 cups chicken stock

- 1 tbsp fish sauce

- 12 oz kelp noodles, rinsed

- ½ cup green onions, chopped

- 2 large eggs, whisked

- Salt and pepper to taste

- 1 cup cooked beef, chopped

- 1 tsp fresh grated ginger

- 1 tsp chopped garlic

- 4 oz shiitake mushrooms, cleansed and sliced

- ¼ cup cilantro, chopped

- Hot sauce for serving

Makes 3 servings

Instructions:

1. Place the chicken in a saucepan and place it over medium heat. Add the fish sauce, kelp noodles, ginger and garlic.

2. Boil for 25 minutes until the kelp is soft. Mix in the eggs and mushrooms. Let it boil for 3 minutes.

3. Adjust the seasoning with salt and pepper. Pour the soup into your bowls and top it with cilantro, beef, green onions and hot sauce.

Coconut Shrimp Soup

Coconut shrimp soup is a nice option if you want to try something different from vegetable soups. This recipe is completely Paleo. It is also low carb and does not contain any dairy.

Ingredients:

- 2 lb raw shrimp, peeled and deveined

- 1 cup onion, diced

- 1 red pepper, diced

- ¼ cup fresh cilantro, chopped

- 1 can coconut milk

- 1 medium lime, juiced

- 2 tbsp coconut oil

- 3 garlic cloves, minced

- 2 jalapenos, diced

- 1 can diced tomatoes

- 1 tbsp chili garlic sauce

- Salt and pepper to taste

Makes 8 servings

Instructions:

1. Place the oil in a large pan. Place it over medium heat and stir until the oil is melted.

2. Cook the onions and peppers for 3 minutes until it is fragrant.

3. Add the shrimps, cilantro, tomato and garlic. Simmer the mixture for 3 minutes and let the flavors infuse.

4. Adjust the seasoning with salt and pepper. Drizzle the lime juice and toss to combine.

No oatmeal cookies

Oatmeal cookies are popular for their rich texture and flavor. These healthier versions are made from flaxseed meal. It has a fresh, chewy and slightly crunchy texture that you will enjoy.

Ingredients:

- 2 cups almond flour

- ½ cup unsweetened shredded coconut

- 1 tsp baking soda

- ½ cup flax seed meal

- 1 tbsp ground cinnamon

- 1 tsp salt

- ¼ cup ghee

- 2 whole eggs

- ¼ cup lard

- ¼ cup date paste

- 1 tsp pure vanilla extract

Add-ons:

- ½ cup dates, chopped

- ½ cup walnuts, chopped

- ½ cup raisins

Makes 24 cookies

Procedure:

1. Set the oven to 375 degrees. Mix the almond flour, unsweetened coconut, baking soda, cinnamon, flax seed meal and salt in a bowl. Stir and whisk until combined.

2. In a separate bowl, add the ghee, lard and date paste. Cream the mixture using a hand mixer. Add the eggs one at a time then whisk thoroughly. Gently add the dry ingredients to the wet ingredients and stir to combine. Add the dates, walnuts and raisins.

3. Line a baking sheet with parchment paper. Drop a small amount of the batter into the pan. Flatten it with a fork. Bake the cookies for 10 minutes then allow to cool for a minute before storing in a container.

Chewy ginger molasses brownies

These chewy brownies can curb your sweet cravings instantly. These cookies are made from natural and Paleo friendly ingredients. Give these cookies a try if you want a break from classic chocolate cookies.

Ingredients:

- 1 cup almond butter

- 2 large eggs, room temperature

- ¾ cup coconut sugar

- 1 tsp baking soda

- ¾ tsp ground cinnamon

- ½ tsp salt

- 3 tbsp molasses

- 2 tsp freshly grated ginger root

- ¼ cup coconut flour

- ½ tsp ginger

- ¼ tsp ground allspice

- Pinch of ground pepper

Makes 25 cookies

Procedure:

1. Cover the pan with parchment paper. Set the oven to 350 degrees.

2. Combine the almond butter, eggs, molasses and ginger in a bowl then whisk together to combine.

3. Sift the coconut sugar, baking soda, cinnamon, coconut flour, ginger, allspice, salt and pepper in a bowl.

4. Slowly incorporate the coconut sugar and spices mixture to the almond butter until combined.

5. Pour it into a wide shallow pan. Make sure that it is about one inch thick only. Bake for 15-25 minutes or until the brownies are done. Let it cool for 10 minutes before slicing.

Zesty Carnival Cake

This beautiful and delicious cake is so easy to make. It is topped with flower petals and bee pollen. You can adjust the sweetness of the frosting by adding more honey and orange juice but if you want a light and semi-sweet frosting, try to follow the quantity stated in the recipe.

Ingredients:

- ½ cup coconut flour plus 2 tbsp more

- ½ tsp baking soda

- 3 whole eggs

- 2 eggs, separated

- 1/3 cup honey

- ¼ tsp salt

- 1 tbsp bee pollen

- ½ cup palm oil

- ¼ cup orange juice

For the frosting:

- 1 tbsp orange juice

- 1 cup palm shortening, cold pressed

- 1 tbsp honey

Garnish:

- Edible flower petals, bee pollen

Makes 8 servings

Procedure:

1. Preheat the oven to 350 degrees.

2. Combine the dry ingredients in a large bowl then set it aside.

3. Separate the egg yolks and set the whites aside.

4. Combine the remaining eggs, red palm oil, orange juice, honey and the two egg yolks. Stir well until well combined.

5. Combine the dry and wet ingredients together. Mix until the batter is smooth.

6. Beat the egg whites until soft peaks form. Add to the batter. Pour the batter into two cake pans.

7. Bake for 35 minutes at 350 degrees. Allow to cool for 10 minutes before placing in the refrigerator.

8. Use a mixer and beat the honey, orange juice and shortening until smooth. Spread the frosting on top of the cake and smooth it out with a spatula.

9. Sprinkle the flower petals and bee pollen on top then chill for an hour before serving.

Conclusion

Thank you again for downloading this book!

I hope this book was able to help you learn more about living gluten free!

The next step is to put this information to use, and begin increasing your health with a gluten free diet!

Finally, if you enjoyed this book, please take the time to share your thoughts and post a review on Amazon. It'd be greatly appreciated!

Thank you and good luck!

www.ingramcontent.com/pod-product-compliance
Lightning Source LLC
Chambersburg PA
CBHW051751050726
47598CB00003B/1428